The Pandemic:
How to Survive & Thrive

TITLE: The Pandemic: How to Survive & Thrive
By: J. K. Morrison
Editor: Angee Costa
Cover Design: Olivia Pro Designs
Copyright 2020

Dedication:

This book is dedicated to my husband, Jesse and my Daughter Alexia. They have been with me through all my business ventures, supporting my ideas and cheering me on every step of the way.

Table of Contents

Foreword

We are entering into a whole new world, with the Coronavirus pandemic upon us. This book will help you and your family stay healthy, feel more at peace, and prepare for the challenges ahead. Some of the text in this book address the early stages of the pandemic. Some countries have since turned the corner. However, the projections are that the virus will be with us for the foreseeable future. There will be multiple waves of the virus, until a vaccine is developed.

We have to sensibly prepare for the emotional, physical, and financial impact of this pandemic. So, congratulations on picking up this book and giving yourself this gift of practical ways to thrive during this or any other global disasters.

This book covers essential topics, including the origin of the novel coronavirus, and how to adjust to a world with the virus. I will offer answers to some of the most fre□uently asked questions about the pandemic and its impact. The contributing author, who is a medical doctor, will share crucial information from a medical perspective. I will show you what you need to know to physically endure a pandemic, including simple ways you can boost your immune system to optimize your health. Equally important is your mental, emotional, and spiritual resilience in these stressful times. I will share techniques to elevate your spirits so that you can navigate life-altering crises. I will discuss how to help family, friends, elderly parents and pets stay sane and safe. I will show you practical ways to take care of those around you.

We will also explore ways to cope with the financial losses that result from this pandemic and simple ways to earn income while at home. Lastly, we will look at how to deal with feelings of trauma when a crisis lingers and interrupts daily life. I will help you set important goals and stay motivated to take needed action in the months ahead. Feel free to skip to chapters more relevant to your current needs and interests.

You will feel empowered and prepared at the end of this book. You will enjoy a sense of greater control in uncertain times so you can thrive even in chaotic times. While the data might sound grim, I want to assure you that there is no need to panic. You have taken appropriate steps to protect yourself by picking up a copy of this book.

Introduction

In 2015, computer mogul, Bill Gates, made a bold prediction. He said:

> *If anything kills over ten million people in the next few decades, it's most likely to be a highly infectious virus rather than a war. Not missiles, but microbes. We are not ready for the next epidemic.*

The evidence supports the above claim. The world had already seen the effects of the swine flu in 2009, Ebola in 2014, and Zika in 2015. We didn't know that a little over four years later, the coronavirus would indiscriminately rip through the globe. COVID-19 has killed hundreds of thousands, sickened millions and devastated financial systems around the world. Lack of preparedness for this pandemic in the USA accounts for the devastation that is sweeping across the country. MERS in 2003 and 2013 put health organizations on notice that there is a host of viruses known as coronaviruses. These clues were missed, trivialized, or ignored. Consequently, we have no vaccines or effective treatments. We essentially forfeited the responsibility to tackle the virus head-on, and the world may be reeling from this for quite a long time.

The Chinese government alerted the world at the end of December 2019, that a "pneumonia of unknown cause" had emerged in Wuhan, located in central China. Approximately a week later, in early January, they reported that the novel (new) coronavirus was the cause of the outbreak. They also reported less than 60 cases and emphasized that there wasn't any evidence of human-to-human spread. Later studies identified the virus as the Severe Acute Respiratory Syndrome Coronavirus 2 (SARS-CoV-2). This strain of SARS-CoV-2 causes the respiratory condition that triggered the pandemic. The virus later became known as COVID-19. World Health Organization (WHO) adopted the name on February 11, 2020. The 'CO' stands for 'corona,' 'VI' for 'virus,' and 'D' for disease. '19' represents the year (2019) the disease first surfaced. The virus was originally referred to as the novel coronavirus, because it had not been previously observed in humans. Human to human transmission of the virus was reported on January, 2020. The degree of infectiousness at incubation seemed unclear, but studies suggested that viral overload in the pharynx was at its peak approximately 4 days post infection, or after onset of symptoms, and declines afterward. The direct and original source of transmission of the virus is still under review. However, because most of the workers at the Wuhan seafood market were the first to be infected, the suggestion is that the strain of virus more than likely, originated from the market. Yet, other research seem to suggest that the virus was introduced by visitors to the market.

Scientists believe bats were most likely the natural reservoir of SARS-CoV-2: meaning that the virus is harbored in the bats for an extended period of time with not pathogenic response. The consensus is that bats are the nevertheless, the source of this family of coronaviruses. For more robust accounts of the origins of the virus, please visit the following websites: the Centres for Disease and Control (CDC) and Public Health England (PHE):

https://www.cdc.gov/coronavirus/2019-ncov/cdcresponse/about-COVID-19.html

https://www.gov.uk/government/publications/wuhan-novel-coronavirus-background-information/wuhan-novel-coronavirus-epidemiology-virology-and-clinical-features#:~:text=On%2031%20December%202019%2C,Hubei%20Province%2C%20China.

The world looks very different during a pandemic. An activity as mundane as going to the supermarket has radically changed in this context. Masks are required to enter buildings, directional signs tell us how to move within the establishments, and registers are cleaned and sanitized after each use. Sporting arenas, theaters, and bowling alleys are closed. Churches have been forced out of the imposing edifices and forced to worship online. No longer can we enter hospitals at will. People who are seriously ill are dropped off at the front door. Grief-stricken relatives say their last goodbyes via Facetime rather than being around dying loved ones.

A survey conducted by the American Enterprise Institute (API) in late May/early June 2020 found that 60% of Americans feared that COVID-19 might strike them and their family members. Responses varied demographically, but 69% of Black Protestants and 42% of white evangelicals were concerned about being infected. While considering the risks involved in returning to regular activity, the majority of Black Protestants

(84%) and Hispanic Catholics (70%) indicated public health was a higher priority. In comparison, a majority of white evangelicals (65%) and white Protestants and white Catholics stated the economy was a more top priority to them.

I believe God gave those in the medical field the intellectual ability to heal. Medical professionals are human and may not always get it right, but we should encourage rather than criticize them. Some pastors remained defiant while still encouraging collective worship. God is a God of order. He certainly is against religious organizations meeting in his name while accelerating infections from COVID-19. This virus requires a common-sense approach. As such most churches have taken to meeting online to minister to their congregations in the wake of lockdown rules. The most useful thing religious organizations can do is continue to pray for an end to the novel coronavirus, for those impacted by the virus, while also praying for renewed knowledge in the field of science and wisdom for physicians. Most people are seizing this period to re-evaluate their relationships with a higher power.

Greetings have also changed in this era where a handshake could transmit the deadly virus. People elbow bump or simply wave from a comfortable six feet. Planes, trains, and automobiles were grounded in March and April of 2020. There was nowhere to go, with everyone sheltering-in-place, The price of fuel plummeted. While most European countries appear to have moved away from complete lockdowns, the United States is still very much in thick of it

There were positive aspects of COVID-19 living, though. People have relearned the value of clean hands, and they are learning the correct way to wash their hands. Another positive is that we have identified the weaknesses in our health systems and supply chains and are working to tighten those processes. The lack of cars on the road reduced greenhouse gas emissions significantly, causing cities from London to Los Angeles and as far off as Beijing to experience smog-free skies for the first time in decades.

All of the world's ecology seems to be enjoying reduced human involvement. Waterways are clearing up and turning blue again, and animals are returning to areas they had abandoned long ago to avoid contact with humans. For example, the canals in Venice are clear and teeming with marine life. Perhaps the most significant benefit of the COVID-19 quarantine is that many have used this time to shift gears and take time out to relax, and spend time with the ones they love. The maddening pace of busy-ness we maintained before the lockdown is just a memory. We are taking time to focus on the crucial things in life.

People have been affected globally. Hardest hit were countries like Italy, Spain, Germany, China, the U. K., the U. S., and Brazil. Most of Europe seems to have turned the corner by lifting some of the lockdowns. Each of these countries have suffered high casualties and heavy financial tolls. However, the U. S. saw a rapid spread of the virus, and the death toll to date stands at approximately 167,000, with one community disproportionately affected: The Black community. The death toll in the U.K. is 46,700 as of August, with black and brown communities taking massive hits. New projections are US casualties hitting 200,000 by November 1, 2020. These numbers may reduce if we all wear masks.

The evidence suggests the coronavirus pandemic disproportionately impacts black and brown communities. Thus, it would help to explore why these disparities exist, and more importantly, how do we address them?

Race and inequality are very complex issues. Thus, it would be problematic to analyze it in simplistic terms. However, health and economics are contributory factors to how the pandemic disproportionately affects people of color:

1. Access to healthcare

Access to healthcare correlates with the capacity to manage crises of the magnitude of COVID-19. Ethnic minorities in the US have the least access to healthcare, are less likely to be insured. Consequently, this creates a deterrence in seeking medical assistance and incurring a bill they may have difficulty paying. On the other hand, the UK provides free healthcare under the National Health System (NHS). However, the statistics regarding access to healthcare appear parallel to the US. Why is that? Studies show that while ethnic minorities in the UK may have free healthcare at their disposal, they are more likely to rank lower on the socio-economic scale. Ethnic minorities are more likely to hold low-paying frontline jobs and have less access to nutritious diets. They are also more likely to live in over-crowded housing, unlike their white counterparts. These same socio-economic issues also plague ethnic minorities in the US, most European countries, and Canada. Ethnic minorities in the USA are less likely to seek medical attention due to a lack of health insurance. In short, poor socio-economic conditions may contribute to co-morbidity factors like obesity, heart disease, and diabetes. These significantly impact infection and fatality from COVID-19. Medical facilities are sparse in more impoverished neighborhoods that are primarily populated by minorities.

2. Frontline exposure:

Ethnic minorities are disproportionately represented in frontline positions. Many are not able to shelter-in-place; neither can they avoid going to work because they rely on the income to feed and care for their families. Studies indicate that many ethnic minorities hold positions in service industries and hospitals that remain open during the worst times of the pandemic. Many of these positions do not offer paid sick leave as a benefit. As a result, workers report to work, even when they might be asymptomatic or ill.

The following is a first-hand account of a COVID-19 survivor and medical professional on the frontlines (his exact words):

"Why did I contract Coronavirus and survive unscathed?"
The answer is simple: To testify to the everlasting presence of one true living God, our father in heaven. I have always prayed with my family every night to thank God for his kindness and goodness, and have consistently asked him to protect us from all dangers, anxiety, and all manner of illness. As we leave our home

everyday we say the rosary. This is routine. My older children, although quite young, have a good understanding of our daily request and prayers to God.

My illness almost raised doubts in my children's faith in God, and a doubt in God's presence and love for us. They asked "why did God abandon us and inflict our dad, with this pestilence?" It was designed to destroy the faith we have in God as a family. Even though I became unwell we prayed fervently to God as usual. When God decides to answer your prayer or deliver you from evil or danger he does it before the danger or evil befalls you.

I became unwell with COVID-19 on Wednesday, 25, March 2020. I woke up feeling rough. It felt like I had been in a fight and had lost woefully. It felt like I had been beaten all over my body, joints, and my eyes with sticks and stones. Shortly afterward, it felt like I had bitten the left side of the back of my tongue, which was very sore. It gradually became painful to swallow. I contacted a colleague. At this point, I suspected I'd contracted the virus and decided to start the process of self-isolation. On day one, I self-isolated in my room from the rest of my family. My meals and water were left outside my door.

As the day progressed, I developed a temperature of 39.8 degrees centigrade with rigors, my muscle ache got worse, and my heart rate, which is normally 70/min had gone up to 98/min. My colleague and I kept in touch always. I started taking pain killers for muscle aches and vitamin C with Zinc. My wife ensured I carried out regular steam inhalation twice a day and provided me with fresh fruits and lots of water to drink regularly and consistently like clockwork. God bless her. I also decided to go out in the garden, with a mask on my face and gloves on hands to exercise for a few minutes daily rather than lying in bed constantly which helped tremendously. However, by day 4, I felt very fragile and exhausted with recurrent fever, chills, and rigors. My left arm felt heavy, and I began to lose my appetite and weight. On that day, I had my first meal at 8 am and could only muster enough energy to eat something small by 8pm that evening. My whole body was hot, weak, with generalized burning sensation and pain, particularly behind my eyes. Something was happening inside of my body. It felt really awful. My heart rate had dropped to roughly 64/min. My test came back positive. After we said our usual night prayer, with me in my room and my family on the other side of my door, I went to bed trusting God.

The next morning I woke up feeling significantly better than I had been the previous day. My fever had come down, my appetite was back, and the muscle aches were gone. I dropped to my knees, praised God, and cried tears of joy. My fever was still present, but I could see that it was gradually diminishing. I kept myself on regularly paracetamol to keep my temperature down. So you see, God delivered me from death so I may fulfill his promise. I am free! I wrote this on April 1, 2020. Please open your ears and eyes to what God has been trying to convey to us all these years. Forgive when you are hurt. This is one of the most important things to do in our daily lives. The Lord's Prayer says, 'forgive us as we forgive those who trespass against us' We all say this prayer regularly but don't always reflect on it. Do away with hatred, wickedness, and envy because these are not of God our father in heaven.

So always remember that God is good, God is love, and God is great, and he truly loves us immeasurably. Make no mistake about that."

This survivor's COVID-19 experience certainly caused me to pause and reflect on the important things in life! It helped me put things in perspective. His faith played a significant role in his recovery. Reading his experience made me appreciate frontline workers and how selfless they are in putting themselves out there to protect us, keep us healthy and alive. God Bless them!

Vitamin D Deficiency and other nutritional concerns

Ethnic minorities sometimes live in conditions that contribute to susceptibility to COVID-19. For example, the lack of quality grocery stores in more impoverished communities results in the absence of healthier nutrition options. Poor nutrition increases the likelihood of chronic health conditions. Many ethnic minorities live in densely populated areas and in close quarters. Coronavirus transmits through close human contact: people who live in cramped conditions are at higher risk of contracting the virus. Living in close quarters makes it impossible to isolate a sick family member, thus potentially exposing other family members to the virus.

You may need to add immune-boosting supplements to your diet. Vitamin D3 is considered an immune booster, and most people who live in colder climates are deficient in Vitamin D3. People of color have higher deficiency levels. The science behind this has been researched and appears conclusive. Current studies point to most individuals needing somewhere between 2000 and 4000 international units per day, depending on medical history. It would be wise to check with your healthcare provider for a specific dosage that fits your circumstances. We will delve deeper into the role vitamin D plays in COVID-19 infections and other chronic medical conditions in the FAQ section of this book.

Vitamin C and zinc are also immune boosters. However, check with your healthcare provider as to whether you can take these supplements.

As the crisis continued to unfold In April 2020, the stats were telling a grave story:

A CDC Morbidity and MortalityWeekly Report (MMWR) report included race and ethnicity data from 580 patients hospitalized with lab-confirmed COVID-19 found that 45% of individuals for whom race or ethnicity data was available were white, compared to 59% of individuals in the surrounding community. However, 33% of hospitalized patients were black compared to 18% in the community and 8% were Hispanic, compared to 14% in the community. This data suggest an overrepresentation of blacks among hospitalized patients.

In short, hospitalizations among black and brown people skyrocketed in comparison to other groups. The death rates in early June were dire.

- Whites were dying at a rate of 45.2 per 100,000.

- Non-black Hispanics/Latinos were dying at the rate of 74.3 per 100,000
- Blacks were dying at a rate of 92.3 per 100,000.

The relationship between ethnic minority communities, particularly people of color and the healthcare industry, is complicated. For some, language barriers present challenges in seeking medical care. Stress is also pervasive among these groups. Living through a pandemic is stressful. Stress wreaks havoc on the immune system, increasing the risk of a viral infection or suffering complications.

Fortunately, there are simple solutions to some of the problems identified in minority communities faced with the challenge of staying healthy during this pandemic.

1. Knowledge is power.

Getting informed about the Coronavirus is the first and most important step people can take to keep themselves and communities healthy. The more informed you about the virus, the better equipped you are to fight the good fight. Avoid urban legends. Get the facts by visiting the CDC, Public Health England (PHE), or the World Health Organization's websites.

2. Eat healthily.

At some point in our journeys, most of us have made promises to ourselves about adopting and sticking to healthier nutritional choices. The presence of a global pandemic is a perfect time to act on and maintain that promise. Most people who are stricken with the virus recover fairly quickly. Nutrition experts advise eating a healthy diet and maintaining a healthy gut for optimum health. For starters, you may want to get into the habit of drinking eight glasses of water daily, ensure half your plate contains fruit and veggies, and stop eating by 8 PM each day. Of course, this may not be suitable for those under special health-related diets requiring snacking after hours.

3. Wash your hands and wear a face mask.

Wearing a face mask when you are around others is a simple and yet effective way to protect them and yourself. You probably have heard the slogan by CNN "A mask can say a lot about who wears it, but even more about the person who doesnt!" When you and those around you wear masks, you protect yourself and others from droplets, which may carry COVID-19 when you talk, cough, or sneeze. You can infect yourself by touching your mouth, nose, and eyes. Washing your hands is considered by most health professionals to be the most critical thing you can do to protect yourself.

4. Contact a doctor if you feel sick.

Call a doctor or 911 (USA) or 111 (UK) if you feel sick. Most healthcare providers prefer that you do not visit their offices or hospitals, but instead call the doctor or a dedicated COVID-19 center to get advice. It is worthy to note that healthcare providers in some European countries are now treating non-COVID related illnesses in their clinics.

5. Keep your stress levels low.

Constantly worrying about your health, family, or finances will not help you and could cause unnecessary harm. You may instead engage in stress-reducing exercise. Connecting with friends and family members helps reduce stress levels.

I leave you with these thoughts concerning your response to the novel coronavirus: How will this impact my family and me in the long run? Now that the panic buying is over, do I still stock up just in case there's a second wave? (the US appears to be knee-deep in the first wave while things seem to have plateaued in the UK). To wear masks or not to wear masks? Should I keep avoiding people? If I get infected, how bad could it get? Could it be fatal? These are valid questions, but if they are dominant in our thought process, why is that? How can we grow spiritually from the effects of COVID 19? Does faith impact our response to this pandemic? Will your faith move you to help others, particularly at times like this, when there's unprecedented hardship? Should we use the lockdowns or partial lockdowns as an excuse not to help, or will we reach out to people, especially those who are feeling a sense of loss? Use this as a call to action to make a difference in these uncertain times.

Chapter 1 - A Whole New World

Visualize yourself going back in time to a week before the terror attacks on September 11, 2001. Knowing what you know today, what would you have done differently? What would be your response if nothing could stop the attack? You would probably first make sure all the people you knew and loved got safely out of New York City or the DC area. Then, you probably would do whatever you could to mentally prepare yourself and the people you love for the challenging days ahead. Finally, you might consider moving some of your money to more secure investment portfolios in light of what was about to happen.

This book will empower and help you prepare psychologically and perhaps financially even while faced with disaster. You can't actually travel back in time, but with the information in this book, you can better prepare yourself for the challenging times amidst this pandemic.

I'm well versed on how people react to dire situations, as a social entrepreneur with a keen interest in the well-being of clients and others. People often bounce back and forth between blame, denial, and complete panic. However, blame, denial, and panic are not effective strategies for dealing with crises. My goal is to show you how to intelligently prepare yourself—and your loved ones—for the emotional, physical, and financial toll of the pandemic.

Just the Facts

What follows is data that might surprise you. My intention is not to alarm you, but to help you during what may be a global disaster like we have never experienced before. It's important to at least be aware of what experts think, since one knows how bad things will get, and no one can accurately predict the future. Experts opine that it is only the beginning of a wave of pandemics the world will face. As we venture into areas unknown to humanity, we expose ourselves to novel diseases for which we have no immunity and for which there are no vaccines or cure. The key is arming ourselves with the facts to be able to combat this virus.

According to many experts:

1. Worldwide, COVID-19 could kill upwards of a million or more. Of course, the development of a vaccine or "treatment" would impact the numbers for the better; efforts to mitigate the spread of the virus will help save lives.

2. The COVID-19 virus kills somewhere between 0.7 and 2.3% of people who contract it—mostly older folks and people with underlying health issues. However, the virus is infecting young, seemingly healthy individuals. Hospitalizations among these groups are on the rise.

3. It could take anywhere between six to nine months to develop a vaccine, but it doesn't end

there. Scores of scientists are racing to develop this coveted vaccine, which promises to not only eliminate the devastating effects of the virus but may provide astronomical profits for the pharmaceutical companies sponsoring the studies. As of early July, a top US pharmaceutical company Novavax was awarded $1.6 billion by the US government to develop a vaccine to combat the novel coronavirus. It was also recently announced that Johnson & Johnson was also awarded $1 billion to develop a vaccine. The two companies are now part of 26 others racing to roll-out a vaccine for COVID-19.

4. People may experience partial immunity to the virus after being vaccinated, as is the case with the flu vaccine. Like most vaccines, there is still that slight chance of getting ill even after being vaccinated.

5. A financial recession or even a depression is likely. Millions of people have already lost their jobs or businesses. Financial markets are already in a panic, and there is little governments can do to stem panic, except bail out companies or provide stimulus checks to citizens.

6. Many hospitals were overwhelmed during the early days of the outbreak due to lack of space and supplies to adequately handle the influx of sick and dying patients. Doctors and hospitals had to make difficult decisions about who lived and who died, as people needed ventilators than were available,

7. A "miracle treatment" may be upon us soon. However, the more likely scenario is people will get sick in "waves." The first wave of Spring was severe, and a Summer 2020 wave is proving to be just as severe. Once people are no longer sheltering in place, additional waves of people will become ill, as is currently the case in the US,

Brazil, China, and now Europe, until we find an effective vaccine. A third wave is possible once the flu season arrives in the fall and winter, and may spark a more drastic resurgence of COVID-19. The US has a fourth of global cases of the novel coronavirus, and yet there's a reluctance at the local level to mandate masks.

A former US health and policy adviser recommended a complete shutdown in July if we are to get a handle on the virus. At the same time, the first phase 3 clinical trial is currently taking place in the US - this is a first of its kind in the US. Other countries like the UK, China, and Brazil have also commenced their trials. The first trial of the Oxford trial was in June, and the first volunteer was a woman from Brazil. Please visit www.ox.ac.uk to get more information on this.

The health and policy adviser cites Spain and Italy as countries shut down for eight weeks early in the pandemic and managed to get their numbers down drastically. However, the US government is calling for a full reopening of schools in fall, while several states continue to experience surges. Experts believe schools may reopen in states with low infection rates but must implement strict guidelines. The CDC was cricicized for not providing sound guidelines; instead, they mention checklists. Meanwhile, school administrators are looking for common sense guidelines on how to reopen schools safely. Some State governors are taking steps to implement stricter guidelines - even partial lockdowns, while others appear to be "playing it by ear." Experts have also concluded that the virus is more contagious and is raging in places with indoor activities, like parties and bars. Beaches appear to be okay, as there are no incidents of people turning up in huge numbers with infections. Testing delays have also gripped parts of the US with medical experts from UCLA warning that aggressive testing is needed. The other problem is that test results are taking too long, with experts stating that a 24-hour turnaround is required to identify clusters and contamination areas before they get out of hand. Most of the infections occur through community spread.

The United Kingdom announced in July that they would impose a 14-day quarantine on travelers from Spain. However, Brits on vacation in Spain note that Spain incidentally has stricter measures than the UK. They also argue that they feel blind-sighted because they weren't forewarned about this before embarking on their trips. Norway has also followed suit and implemented a two-week quarantine on travelers from Spain. The UK recently imposed a 14-day quarantine on travelers from France. This sent British vacationers into a frenzy, while trying to beat the deadline to make it back in the country.

The following is a first-hand account of a COVID-19 survivor in the UK (her exact words) :

"On March 10th, my daughter informed me that she wasn't feeling well. She had a cough and a fever. I asked her to call NHS 111, the dedicated line for COVID-19. She did, relayed her symptoms and answered a number of their questions. Not being high risk and young, she was advised to monitor the symptoms. I gave her paracetamol and a lot of water: the two most important things to keep the temperature down and stay hydrated.

Then on the 12th, I had a meeting which finished at 10 pm and on my way back I thought it too late to cook anything, then decided to buy fish and chips; I usually don't eat much fast food. On getting home, after consuming a few mouthfuls, my stomach turned and started hurting that I decided to throw the rest in the bin. I considered the oil it was fried in, because I reacted, or my stomach has become sensitive to fast food. On the way back to my room, I told my daughter that I wasn't feeling too good and was going to lie down for a bit. I slept off and woke up in the morning with temperature, fever, and diarrhea. I started taking paracetamol, drinking a lot of water, and Vitamin C with Zinc.

I got progressively worse throughout the weekend, and by Monday, I could not move. It felt like I had been in a battle with two Mike Tysons, and beaten to a pulp. My daughter, at this time, had bounced back and was looking after me. I called NHS 111, gave them my symptoms, answered their questions: they sent an ambulance. They arrived, ran checks, and recommended I went to the hospital. On asking whether I would be tested in hospital, they said no; I refused to go as I did not want to expose myself even more to the virus. My GP agreed with me, and the paramedics advised us to call 999 if it got worse. I was diligent with taking the right doses of paracetamol at the proper intervals and was able to bring down the high temperature and suppress the fever. However, the migraine continued; my eyes, ears, and ribcage were hurting, had dizzy spells, and lost my taste and appetite. My breathing got worse. Since I had never had respiratory problems, it was a new sensation that I could not manage. I guess I panicked and, in so doing, worsened my case. At this time, I was so tired that I could not speak. My daughter had to make the second call to 999, informing them of my worsening state. The paramedics came out again for observation and decided that, although I was feeling terrible, I could not go to the hospital because there were cases worse than mine; the NHS was overwhelmed - and by their third visit, I decided that this was now between God and I. I started taking brewed ginger, garlic, hibiscus, orange, lime, and lemon, sweetened with honey; I said a lot of prayers. Friends and family were doing the same. I had a lot of silent conversations with

God. One thing I did right from the beginning was steam inhalation with drops of vicks or olbas oil. I had hot baths with lavender and bath salts. Helped me sleep better. I also used a humidifier to aid my breathing. By the 15th day, I could now sit up in bed, which marked the start of my recovery journey. One thing this illness does is sap your energy. It took almost a week to build it back up to even venture down the stairs. I am glad to say that I have recovered and full of energy. I have carried on with taking all the natural remedies and vitamins. I have been on daily Vitamin D for the past four years, which I suppose helped my immune system.

It is necessary to fully rest and worry about nothing and vital to catch the virus around the nasal region and throat before it descends to the lungs. Applying heat helps, hence the steam inhalation and drinking anything hot.

The lesson so far is that there are varied symptoms, and not everyone will experience the same. The list of symptoms keeps growing daily. There is nothing gradual about the illness, and the deterioration rate is rapid. Some people did not even have enough time to write their wills or make peace. No time to come to terms with what's happening to you. Viral overload is real, and I believe the level of exposure determines the severity; hence the reason we must socially isolate, stay home, and only go out when it is essential.

Since there is no known cure or vaccine, having a healthy immune system is the guaranteed way of standing a chance to fight it. That is, of course, assuming there are no other underlining illnesses. If taking Vitamin C, make sure that it is with Zinc for absorption. I suggest that if your daily activity doesn't include at least 30 minutes of getting direct sunshine, best between 12 and 3 pm, then start taking Vitamin D supplements, which help the immune system. I know people in sweltering climates who are deficient in Vitamin D. It is a SUPER vitamin vital for brainwork, immunity, strong bones etc,. Then lots of fruits high in vitamin C and vegetables.

Lastly, my faith was my anchor and hope, and being Lenten season; I saw the illness as a trial that I would overcome by His Grace. I thank God for His mercies and Faithfulness and continue to pray for His protection for ALL.

A close friend also shared her COVID-19 experience with me. She is a Community Officer with London Metropolitan Police in the UK. She realized she might have contracted the virus when she couldn't smell a Class B drug while on patrol. She found out at the same time that she had lost her sense of taste. She became naturally alarmed but continued to monitor her symptoms. Thankfully, she didn't develop any other severe symptoms and was able to carry on working. Her symptoms lasted eight days. On the other hand, her daughter had the same symptoms, but hers lasted for seven weeks. She worked from home. My theory is that my friend's symptoms were shorter than her daughter's because she continued to be active, as is required by her job, which entails walking for miles on patrol.

Things can evolve quickly, despite projections by the experts. The good news is, once an effective vaccine is developed, financial markets and jobs will start the recovery process.

The best defense under the current circumstances is to be physically, emotionally, and spiritually prepared as best as you can. When the normal rules governing daily life are disrupted (think the 2008 financial crash), people get panicky and financial markets go into a frenzy. However, once we have adequate information, tools, and the right perspective, we quickly learn to adjust to a new world, albeit operating under new rules.

Former U.S. President Franklin Delano Roosevelt once famously said, "The only thing we have to fear is fear itself." Fear and panic can create reckless behavior. For example, during the early stages of the pandemic, a fearful friend bought a bottle of hand sanitizer on Amazon for $30. I bought five bottles of a comparable brand at the local dollar store for $5. Fear can lead to bad financial decisions, which can impact stress levels.

Read this book; Do not to succumb to fear. Remember, you are not in this alone! Not only is the whole world dealing with this pandemic (so you're in good company even if you're home alone), and historically, we have survived tougher times.

History demonstrates that the human race is a resilient species. We adjust to a new normal fairly quickly, after initial fear and panic. We somewhat resume our routine after that initial wave of panic. The toughest phase of a crisis is not knowing what lies ahead—what I call "living with uncertainty." I will discuss specific methods for handling fear and uncertainty, in later chapters.

So, welcome to this new world with new rules for thriving. Now let's get into the specifics of how best to handle the unusual times ahead.

Chapter 2 - Quick FAQs regarding the Virus

Data on the coronavirus pandemic changes rapidly. Therefore, answers to frequently asked questions reflected below may have changed by the time you read this. However, this book includes answers to commonly asked questions which will be relevant for some time. You may also utilize google, or go to the FAQ sections of the U.S.'s Centers for Disease Control, the U.K.'s National Health Service, UK's Public Health England (PHE) and the World Health Organization websites. You may also access those sites here:

https://www.cdc.gov/coronavirus/2019ncov/index.html

https://www.nhs.uk/conditions/coronavirus-covid-19/

https://www.who.int/emergencies/diseases/novel
-coronavirus-2019.

https://www.gov.uk/government/publications/cor
onavirus-outbreak-faqs-what-you-can-and-cant-

https://www.canada.ca/en/public-
health/services/diseases/2019-novel-
coronavirus-infection.html?topic=tilelink

Here are frequently asked questions (FAQs) and
answers.

**What is a virus? How does it impact human
cells, and how does it spread?**

Mr. Vincent Kika, an NHS Emergency Room
Consultant/Physician in London, offers the
following explanation on viruses and how they
impact cells: *A cell is a living thing made up of
lipids, proteins, carbohydrates, enzymes, and
DNA as well as other functioning parts within the
cell required to keep the cell alive and of course
our whole being. DNA and RNA are compounds*

that hold our genetic blueprint. They hold instructions on how and what our cells should make, such as proteins for the cell structure and other vital functions that cells need to stay healthy and alive.

On the other hand, a virus is not a living thing but is made up of a protein, lipid, and carbohydrate coat, which envelopes a DNA or an RNA all put together without any real functioning parts found in a cell. Thus, viruses do not have enzymes like living cells do and, do not have a cellular structure or function. However, when they come in contact with a cell, they start behaving like a living thing and essentially take over the cell's function.

Viruses may have originated and evolved from bits of DNA of some animals. However, as proteins, lipids, and carbohydrates that make up a virus occur naturally, a virus can be put together in a lab with the right facilities. Viruses need cells to multiply and are unable to cause harm or injury until they infect a living cell and poison it. Hence the name virus in Latin means poison or venom.

Once a virus comes in contact with a healthy cell, it essentially hijacks the cell function and poisons it by using the cell's DNA to make its proteins and several copies of its DNA or RNA. The process confuses the cell and takes over the cell's regular function required to stay healthy. The virus then gives the cell instructions to replicate and form more viruses, which then infect more healthy cells, rendering them useless to the body. This process of multiplication within cells and the inability for the infected cell to carry out its survival functions and grow as it should, results in 1) cell damage, 2) change in the architecture of the cell or, 3) death of the cell and, 4) unfortunately sometimes the death of the person whose cells are infected by the virus. The Pandemic Survival Guide contains information to simplify the complex COVID-19 "terrain." The book should allay your fears and anxieties and prepare and guide you to cope with the pandemic. The virus typically spreads via person-to-person transmission when people are in proximity with one another and through respiratory droplets emitted while coughing, sneezing and, in rare cases, talking. Droplets are inhaled through the nostrils and possibly migrate to the lungs. Studies indicate that asymptomatic people routinely spread COVID-19. However, wearing N95 masks or other effective masks (Pls go to CDC or WHO website to obtain current recommendations on masks) sometimes protects others from contracting the virus from asymptomatic individuals.

Will Vitamin D protect me from contracting COVID-19?

According to Mr. Kika, MD, "Vitamin D plays a vital role in the body's immune function; it is integral to the prevention of bacterial infections and viral infections that cause colds, the flu, and acute respiratory infections such as those caused by COVID-19. It is also essential in preventing other debilitating diseases such as diabetes, cancer, etc. Evidence suggests that COVID-19 infection can is preventable by taking vitamin D supplements.

"The suggested dose for black people and other people of color is at least 400 units (10 mcg) to 800 units (20mcg) per day, particularly those who live in temperate parts of the world and do not get enough sunshine throughout the year. This dose should be nearer the 800 (20mcg) - 1000 (25mcg) unit dosage, particularly in winter or in summer, when not exposed to enough

sunlight as a result of working indoors all day long. The above dosage information is not shared as medical advice. Therefore, please consult your doctor before you commence vitamin D supplementation.

Why are older people, black people, and other people of color more prone to contracting COVID-19?

Socio-economic factors, over-crowded accommodation, pre-existing illness in COVID-19 positive patients such as renal failure, diabetes, hypertension etc., have all been implicated. These factors are worth considering as potential reasons people of color or black people, and the elderly are more affected by COVID-19. The data motivated me to conduct evidence-based research with particular reference to vitamin D.

Synthesization of vitamin D into the skin occurs with exposure to sunlight; it is in a diet rich in oily fish and shellfish. Cod liver oil is also a great source of Vitamin D. Most of us require additional amounts from our food or from supplements to maintain adequate levels. Receptors for vitamin D are present in all cells of the body. Vitamin D helps the body fight off infections and provides other protective benefits - against bone diseases such as rickets and other conditions such as diabetes and Alzheimers. We know that COVID-19 is primarily a respiratory tract infection. Therefore, respiratory tract infections are avoidable by taking daily, and weekly doses of vitamin D. Black people and other people of color have more melanin pigmentation. This pigmentation determines skin tone.

Melanin protects us against sunburn and skin cancer. Still, unfortunately, it prevents us from absorbing adequate amounts of sunshine necessary to produce optimal levels of vitamin D. This is true all year round in temperate climates, like the UK and some parts of the USA. Up to 40% of the UK population is vitamin D deficient during colder months. This number is nearer the 45% mark in the USA.

People who live around the equator in Africa have adequate vitamin D production. The proper production of the vitamin explains the low infection rates of COVID-19 in that region, such as, in Nigeria near the equator. The optimal production of vitamin D in people who live in that region is explainable by the high intensity of the sun around the equator.

Caucasians, on the other hand, can absorb vitamin D in more copious amounts because they possess less melanin. However, a Caucasian who uses sunscreen, lacks enough sun exposure, and dietary supplements will succumb to infections just as easily as a black person of a person of color. The same is true for the elderly who are inactive and confined indoors. The recommendation is to increase exposure to sunlight, eat a diet rich in vitamin D, or take vitamin D supplements. If you decide to take a vitamin D supplement, choose one that contains D3 (cholecalciferol). Please note that the dosage information below is not shared as medical advice. Therefore, consult a healthcare provider before you commence vitamin D supplementation. It may also be advisable to discuss checking your levels with your healthcare provider.

Vitamin D comes in different strengths. Commonly as
- *400 units which is equivalent to 10 mcg*
- *500 units which is equivalent to 12.5 mcg*
- *800 units which is equivalent to 20 mcg*
- *1000 units which is equivalent to 25 mcg*

- *And other strengths*

You might see the dose displayed as i.u (i.u stands for international units)

British National Formulary (BNF) and Public Health England (PHE) recommended daily dose of vitamin D:

1. *For the prevention of Vitamin D deficiency.*
   ADULTS: 400 units per day
   CHILDREN: 400 units per day
For black people and people of color (adults) consider doubling this dose daily particularly in winter months
2. *For the treatment of Vitamin D deficiency.*
   ADULTS: 800 units (which is roughly equivalent to about 20 mcg) per day
   CHILDREN: nothing written for treatment in children."
   Check with your healthcare provider to ensure it is safe for you to take Vitamin D supplements.

Should I wear a face mask?

The debate at the onset of the pandemic was whether wearing a mask effectively curbed the spread of the novel coronavirus. The consensus was that wearing a mask does not reduce the chances of a healthy person being exposed to and becoming infected with COVID, but that wearing a mask lowers the risk of spreading the virus through droplets while talking, coughing and sneezing. Research shows that masks protect those who are COVID-19 free from potentially being exposed and infected.

Wearing a mask is a sensible way to protect yourself and people around you. Wearing a mask is advisable even if you are not sick, contrary to reports at the beginning of the pandemic. While the CDC suggested that the most effective mask to wear is the N95 respirator, other sources cite the use of surgical masks, cloth masks, ski masks, and makeshift masks made out of anything from bandanas to scarves as being better than not using a mask at all. Wearing a mask can also prevent you from touching your mouth and nose; the virus is often transmitted by touching one's face with one's hand.

According to experts at the San Francisco General Hospital, masks are necessary now and will be for the foreseeable future. They opine that we need to get used to wearing masks as we fight through this pandemic. The Chinese population and indeed most of Asia was already used to wearing masks. A habit necessitated by the 2002/2003 SARS outbreak which sickened 8000 and killed approximately 800, before it was successfully controlled. Thus, it was customary for people in Asia to wear masks prior to the outbreak. Top infectious disease specialists all agree that there isn't evidence that suggests that masks are harmful to humans. They recommend wearing what feels comfortable for you. The emphasis is on protection of others and prevention of the disease.

Is it safe to shop for groceries?

Research shows that sanitizing shopping cart handles before use, using credit cards or contactless payment instead of cash-handling, or shopping after rush hour to avoid crowded areas are significant precautionary measures. Wearing a mask while shopping and washing hands or using hand sanitizer after handling items at the grocery store are good safety practices. Remember to wear a mask when in crowded areas.

How do I know if I need to self- quarantine?

The Centers for Disease Control and Prevention (CDC) and Public Health England (PHE) recommend a 14-day self-quarantine (self-isolation) should a family member test positive. If you or your family member have a fever, dry cough, or shortness of breath, contact your healthcare provider or a dedicated COVID-19 center immediately if the symptoms are mild, self-quarantine until you have been symptom-free 14 days. Your healthcare provider would be in the best position to tell you your options if you have underlying health conditions.

Who is most at risk?

Everyone in the following groups is at a higher risk: elderly family members and friends, people with underlying health conditions, and those who immunocompromised. Recent research suggests that being overweight is a significant factor in COVID-19 morbidity.

Can I contract COVID-19 from food?

Experts believe that the virus is not likely to be transmitted by food. The CDC conducts studies on food-borne and waterborne illnesses and emphatically state that COVID-19 is not "food-borne-driven or food-service driven." The virus is a person-to-person respiratory disease. The virus is spread mostly through respiratory droplets from an infected person. The modes of transmission are coughing, sneezing, or talking within 6 feet of another individual. The CDC recommends wearing masks, social distancing, and washing hands regularly to prevent the spread. However, the CDC opined that you could get the virus from contaminated surface, and touching one's face. Again, the recommendation is hand-washing with soap and water for 20 seconds and wiping surfaces with anti-viral solutions.

Can I get it from shipped packages including, packaged food?

According to WHO, the virus is unlikely to persist after shipping. The health organization says science doesn't support the idea that transmission occurs within the food chain or food packaging. They urge people not to fear food, food packaging, and food delivery. It is highly unlikely that the virus will stay alive and active on a package after being exposed to different conditions and temperatures. If that still doesn't provide solace, a virologist from an Ivy League university in the USA states that even if the virus comes in contact with food, the stomach acids will kill the virus once it's in the digestive tract.

Is there a cure?

Not yet! Those who contract the virus receive support to alleviate symptoms. Supportive care means taking measures to address your symptoms so you can feel as comfortable as possible.

Do pneumonia shots protect against Covid-19?

Per former CDC Chief Medical Officer, pneumonia shots do not prevent COVID-19 induced pneumonia

What if I test for COVID-19 and get a negative result?

A negative test indicator doesn't necessarily mean the patient isn't infected. Approximately 10-30% of test results come back negative even when the person tested has the disease.

Therefore, if you have symptoms, get tested at least twice.

Can pets spread COVID-19?

CDC studies suggest that the risk of animals spreading the virus to humans is low. COVID-19 was confirmed in a cat in the UK. The cat fully recovered. Veterinary experts suggest that the cat may have contracted the disease from someone who tested positive within the household. Experts believe the virus is unlikely to pass from pets to humans, albeit that there have been human-to-pet infections,

How worried should I be about getting sick?

Everyone should equally share concerns about potential infection. People 60 and over are most at risk of infection. People with underlying health conditions such as diabetes, chronic lung disease, and chronic kidney disease are at risk of infection: chronic liver disease, most types of cardiovascular diseases, active cancers, and immuno-compromised people are also at risk of infection. However, current studies show that young people are just as vulnerable.

What should I do if I feel sick?

Contact your healthcare professional or dedicated COVID-19 center to report your symptoms. If you do not have a Family Physician, General Practitioner, or any healthcare provider, contact your local urgent care or emergency department for medical advice. The CDC and PHE recommend self-quarantine (self-isolation) if someone came in contact with the virus. Self-isolation refers to separating infected persons from those who are free of the virus. You may check out CDC webpage on this FAQ and the next FAQ:

https://www.cdc.gov/coronavirus/2019-ncov/if-you-are-sick/quarantine.html?CDC_AA_refVal=https%3A%2F%2Fwww.cdc.gov%2Fcoronavirus%2F2019-ncov%2Fif-you-are-sick%2Fquarantine-isolation.html

https://www.gov.uk/coronavirus?gclid=EAIaIQobChMItNiBkJmJ6wIVwu3tCh1t9g17EAAYASAAEgLAfvD_BwE

What if somebody in my household gets infected?

Family members who contract the virus and do not have life-threatening symptoms should be cared for at home while following guidelines provided by the Centers for Disease and Control and Public Health England. Infected family members should isolate in separate rooms and bathrooms to minimize contact with the rest of the family. Communal areas should have adequate airflow with open windows. Visitors should not be allowed, except those who have to be there for a purpose.

Infected family member(s) should wear face masks when in contact with healthy family members. Healthy family members may consider wearing masks while their family member remains unwell. Wearing masks reduces the likelihood of infection. Sanitize household items used by sick family member(s). Remember to wash your hands frequently.

How do I get tested?

The CDC recommends calling your healthcare provider if you think you have been exposed or are experiencing symptoms related to COVID-19. PHE also recommends testing if you have symptoms suggestive of COVID-19 infection at a test site near you or with a home test kit. The ultimate decision on whether you should be tested lies with medical professionals. It is essential to note that, not everyone who contracts the virus gets tested. Obstacles to testing currently range from a scarcity of testing kits to an asymptomatic person requesting testing. In other words, there is a chance you may not be a candidate for testing, even if you think you are. Various companies are manufacturing tests at a rapid rate. Thus, those who need tests in the future stand a good chance of getting tested.

How is the virus different from the flu?

Some symptoms of COVID-19 are similar to those of the flu - dry cough, fever, shortness of breath, and general malaise. However, there are notable differences. Doctors try to rule out the flu at the outset, given the similarities between both. Spring allergy season triggers similar symptoms, adding a diagnostic wrinkle to an already challenging situation. The flu differs from COVID-19 because there is a vaccine for the flu and no vaccine yet for COVID-19. The flu killed 64,000 in the USA over 12 months; as of August 2020, there are 170,000 COVID-19 deaths over five months in the USA. The US is averaging 1,000 deaths per day as of August 17. Therefore, until there is a cure, COVID-19 is more lethal than the flu.

Is it advisable to go to the park?

Yes! Exercise is a significant boost to the immune system. Outside activity is an alternative to exposing oneself to the gym, where high-contact equipment pose considerable risk of infection. Scientific research shows that infectious germs live on surfaces at the gym for a substantial length of time. This information is crucial in light of medical evidence that time plus the virus presents a high probability of infection.

My children are scared. What can I tell them?

One of the most important things to do during these trying times is to find ways to manage our anxiety before addressing our children's concerns. The most meaningful way to address those concerns is to listen to them and provide reassurance. Refrain from making dismissive statements such as, "It'll be fine." Such dismissive responses evoke feelings of not being heard, which can do more harm than good at times, such as these. Stress importance of hand-washing before and after meals, and after using the bathroom. Children (and adults) should sing the "Happy Birthday Song" twice while hand-washing to ensure the elimination of all pathogens. School closures should be conveyed in a positive light to children, given that it creates quality time with the family — a time to engage in fun activities as a family. Children (and adults) should be encouraged to stay active while adhering to social distancing rules.

Is it advisable to order delivery during a pandemic?

While staying indoors is recommended, it is also a fact that we need food and other pertinent items for survival. However, how can you remain protected while ensuring the delivery drivers are protected? Delivery makes sense for the elderly and those with chronic health issues. Ultimately, online delivery is an excellent resource for sheltering at home and a way to keep businesses running and profitable. You may also want to think about tipping delivery drivers who risk their health to serve others. It is advisable to wipe down delivery bags and outer casing of boxes or containers with anti-viral wipes.

Is air travel safe?

Germs are not easily transmitted in aircrafts because of the air circulation and filtration systems. However, bear in mind that social distancing may be difficult on crowded airplanes. On the bright, side, I know people who have traveled transatlantic and did not contract the virus. Most airport authorities conduct temperature checks upon arrival to determine possible infection.

Can I send my children back to school?

The decision is a personal one and varies from country to country. It is handled at the local level in some countries. I polled parents in the US and the UK, and the responses varied from a lack of comfortability to the jury is still out and the affirmative. Still, countries like Denmark seem to have had success implementing a safe back to school policy.

Should I ride the subway or underground?

This decision is personal and is a question of risk tolerance. Countries urge citizens to continue riding while adhering to social distancing rules. Seeking alternate forms of travel may be wise at this point. However, if this is not an option for you, do ride with caution. The science is inconclusive about how long the virus can live and remain transmittable on surfaces. If you must ride the subway, take such steps as avoiding overcrowded cars, wear disposable gloves while holding on to poles and discard as soon as you exit the subway. In the event you do not have gloves or don't want to wear gloves, hand-sanitizers will suffice. Avoid touching your face and always wash your hands upon returning home. Always dispose of gloves and masks in trash cans instead of dropping them on the street where they are a hazard to people who clean sidewalks.

What makes the COVID-19 outbreak so different?

There's currently no universally accepted treatment or cure for COVID-19. However, pharmaceutical companies and scientists are still studying and gathering data to create safe pharmaceutic drugs or a vaccine to tackle this virus. Data indicates that it is more lethal than the flu, but studies are inconclusive. Additionally, the elderly and those with underlying medical conditions are particularly at risk. Please visit the following website to get answers to COVID-19 questions, as reported by CNN:

https://edition.cnn.com/audio/podcasts/coronavirus-questions-and-answers

Chapter 3 - Physical Preparation for You and Your Loved Ones

The USA and to a lesser extent, the UK are still battling phase 1 of the Coronavirus. While the USA seemed to be turning the corner, things have taken a turn for the worse. Thirty-two states report a spike in cases. Thus, the battle may continue for a while longer in the USA. The UK and other European countries appear to have turned the corner. However, this may be suspect since current data suggests that the virus typically stages a comeback once rules are relaxed.

There were surges in Leicester in the UK, Florida, Texas, and Arizona in the USA, and recently in Spain and France. Some of these areas went back to lockdown, while others simply tightened the rules. The problem is, most people are having a hard time embracing what will be our new normal for a while. It is critical in light of recent data, to be prepared with what you will physically need to survive and thrive. You may have noticed that when the fear of this pandemic really "hit," there was a scarcity of items such as hand sanitizers, water, lysol/dettol spray, toilet paper, and pasta. One day toilet paper was everywhere, and the next day people were stealing it from the hands of old ladies at Costco. Things evolved fast. The good news is, shortages of supplies do not last long, based on what happened in China. Somehow, even in the Wuhan province where the virus began and a complete lockdown was enforced, people still managed to get food, water, and toilet paper. So, there is no need to hoard such items. On the other hand, there are common-sense things you can do to physically prepare your family for the challenging times ahead

It's always a good idea to prepare for eventualities. Having, a short-term supply of basics is a smart move. See the following guidelines:

Home Preparation:

While food and water will likely be widely available, it's always a good idea to prepare. Having, a short-term supply of basics, is a smart move.

Water

At a minimum, a three-day supply of water per individual is advisable. A week's supply would be ideal.

- ➢ A gallon per person per day for consumption and sanitation.
- ➢ Minors, new mothers, and the sick may need more water.
- ➢ Individuals who live in warmer climates may need more water.

> Water should be stored tightly in sanitary non-pvc containers.

Food:

> A two-week supply of non-perishable foods for each member of your household. This is necessary should you get sick and need to self-☐uarantine.

> Select foods requiring minimal preparation with water; Purchase a manual can opener if you don't already have one.

> Purchase readily consumable canned goods, vegetables, beans, and fruits, such as:

☐ Oats or other grains

☐ Protein or fruit bars

☐ Nuts

☐ Peanut butter

☐ Rice

☐ Dried fruit

☐ Beans and lentils

☐ Canned Juices and Coffee (optional)

☐ Non-perishable pasteurized milk

☐ Food for infants

☐ Fresh frozen veggies and fruits

☐ Oats or other grains

☐ Comfort/stress foods

Nose and Mouth Protection:

You may notice people wearing different types of masks. Depending on what you read, these masks are either not helpful or potentially lifesaving. Masks are useful and even necessary in the fight against COVID-19. Masks labeled as N95 are effective in preventing the coronavirus. However, people must wear them correctly. Fortunately, N95 masks are not as scarce as they were at the beginning of the pandemic. However, healthcare professionals are prioritized for personal protection equipment, such as masks. Surgical masks, cloth masks, and even makeshift masks are ideal for protecting droplets that may carry the virus. Masks is they keep you from touching your face. Hand-to-face contact is perhaps the most common form of transmission of the virus.

The average person touches his or her face about 22 times each hour. Who knew? I quickly learned that my hands are absolutely in love with my face. Therefore, if you go outside and have any contact with potentially sick people, please consider facial protection, as well as gloves.

Soap and Hand Sanitizer:

Fortunately, after a brief period of panic-buying, soap and hand sanitizers are now more available to purchase than they were at the start of the pandemic. An alternative to hand-sanitizers is 91% rubbing alcohol combined with Aloe Vera gel to create your own hand sanitizer. The important thing is to get in the habit of washing your hands thoroughly with warm water for 20 seconds several times a day. Twenty seconds is the e☐uivalent of singing the "Happy Birthday song" twice. Consider singing out loud just to give you a reason to smile despite what is going on.

A great way to use hand sanitizer is to get a little bottle of it, and clip it or string it directly to your belt or pants, particularly when you leave your house. Sanitize your hands immediately after purchasing groceries, touching counters, or just about anything outside your house. Your smartphone is easy to contaminate, so wiping down your smartphone periodically with a disinfectant wipe, rubbing alcohol, or hand sanitizer is a good idea.

The Air You Breathe

According to the CDC, air purifiers with HEPA filters provide additional protection, if the virus is airborne in your home. The Coronavirus can stay airborne (for example if someone sneezes) for an approximate half-hour. As a general matter, air purifiers also make the air healthier in the home. Thus, an air purifier with a HEPA filter is an excellent investment in a time such as this.

First Aid Kit

A basic First Aid Kit is essential at a time like this when hospitals are likely to be overwhelmed with cases.   More importantly, hospitals, GP's surgeries, and doctor's offices are places which should be avoided during this crisis. Learning first aid at a time like this would make a difference during an emergency. Thus, consider embarking on an online first aid class. However, owning the following items is a great start.

Recommended items:

☐ Latex gloves: (if you have an allergy to latex consider other sterile gloves).

☐ Adhesive bandages in a variety of sizes.

☐ Sterile dressing in case of bleeding

☐ Cleansing agent/ and antibiotic towelettes for disinfecting wounds.

☐ Thermometer

☐ Ointment to prevent infection from possible burns.

☐ Optical solution to flush the eyes or as a general decontaminant.

☐ Antibiotic ointment to prevent infection

☐ Prescription medication such as insulin, inhalers, and EpiPen. Other medical supplies such as blood pressure and blood sugar monitors.

☐ Nonprescription medication:

☐ Potassium Iodide

☐ Aspirin, Tylenol, Paracetamol, or pain relievers in the same category.

☐ Antidiarrhea medication

☐ Antacid (for upset stomach)

☐ Prescription Drugs:

Have at least a month's supply of prescription medication on hand for family members who need them.

Special Needs Items:

Family members with special needs require planning as everyone else, and sometimes more, to be prepared for pandemic-induced illness.

Babies will need the following:

- Formula
- Bottles
- Diapers
- Powdered milk
- Medication
- Diaper rash ointment
- Moist Towelettes

Adults:

- Prescription drugs
- Dentures, if applicable

- Contact lenses and other optical supplies
- Supplemental eyewear

Additional supplies for Seniors:

- An inventory of prescription medication including dosage. Include allergy information

- Extra eyeglasses and batteries or hearing aids.

- Extra batteries for wheelchairs or other supply kit.

- Emergency supply kit should include a list of identifying serial numbers to medical devices such as blood sugar monitors

- Health insurance cards

- List of medical providers with emergency contacts.

Persons with Disabilities:

- Support systems are invaluable during emergency.

- A trusted member of the support network should be entrusted with the keys to your dwelling, or consider installing a key-safe installed outside your door.

- Lastly, purchase a battery-operated radio to stay abreast of pertinent information, should you be faced with a power outage.

Taking the steps discussed in this chapter will adequately prepare you for the challenges ahead; you'll be better prepared mentally and emotionally.

Chapter 4 - Taking Care of Your Health

Taking excellent care of your health is your best defense against COVID-19, in addition to taking care of dependents (kids, mates, parents, pets). Stress, fear, and uncertainty may be our daily companions for a while. Coronavirus is not our only enemy. According to the American Medical Association, 80 to 90% of all disease is stress-related. It is imperative to develop coping strategies for handling stress-related fear.

Managing anxiety and fear is not a one-time event, but an ongoing, even lifelong process. One of the most effective ways to fight stress is to interrupt worrying thoughts patterns at least once an hour. Therefore, I will share techniques to manage stress that take just a minute or two each to do. You can improve your health and boost you immunity by engaging in these simple techniques. Taking such steps help tap into a clearer state of mind, and equips you better to handle the pandemic or other challenging situations. I go into more detail on how to combat fear, in the next chapter; but for now, the following could be of immediate help.

One Minute Stress Reduction (by: Psychotherpist, Jonathan Robinson)

"First, stand up and shake your entire body. Begin by shaking both your arms, then each leg—one at a time. Move your shoulders, an area where we hold a lot of tension. Then relax your jaws. Finally, motion up and down on your toes for thirty seconds while your body shakes loose. This motion will help to boost your immune system, get your energy going, and help you overcome feelings of fear and being overwhelmed. It works surprisingly well. Take the utmost care while engaging in the moves to prevent injury. Ensure you also check with your healthcare provider about participating in these

simple exercises if you have underlying health conditions.

Another quick method for overcoming stress is something I call "The Two Minute Love Meditation." This technique requires you to think of a person, child, or pet who you have great affection for. This simple method reduces cortisol levels in the body for up to five and a half hours, besides quieting your mind, in less than two minutes. Here are the four easy steps:

1. *Close your eyes, take a very deep breath, hold it for 10 seconds, then exhale with a sigh as you focus on the sensations in your chest.*

2. *Picture or think of someone you really care about. It could be a mate, friend, child, or a pet (babies and pets are great). Imagine them giving you a look that reminds you how much you care about them.*

3. *Think about how much you appreciate this person or pet; think of good times you've shared, and how grateful you are that they are in your life.*

4. *You can imagine holding or hugging the one you love. After a minute or two, slowly open your eyes and enjoy the feeling of peace and calm.*

This simple method, if practiced regularly, can help you go from stressed out to blissed out in under two minutes. Studies show that it actually changes your brain waves and and relaxes your nerves, effectively interrupting the momentum of anxiety people can get caught up in. This simple tool can help you to keep your sanity when faced with the immense stress and the uncertainty of disasters."

Do whatever you can to maximize your health and your immune response systems, including managing stress. You've probably heard the basics a hundred times, but for easy reference, here are the commonsense ways of making sure you stay in good health:

- Eat a diet mostly consisting of fruits and vegetables.

- Get 7 to 9 hours of sleep each night. Very important!

- Avoid processed foods and high amounts of sugar which all decrease immunity to disease.

- Experts believe taking the following immune-boosting vitamins: Vitamin D3 and Vitamin C with Zinc are an excellent defense against the coronavirus (Check with your healthcare provider)

- Exercise a minimum of three times a week for a minimum of thirty minutes each time (or if doing high-intensity workouts, you need only about ten minutes). Consult your healthcare provider if you have health concerns or underlying health issues that would prohibit you from engaging in physical activity.

Exercise

Studies show that exercise boosts the immune system, and sometimes lessens the severity of symptoms. I exercise routinely. I will share tips that can make exercising (without going to a gym) fun and effective.

Let me ask you a question at the outset: What is the best exercise? A lot of people think it's walking, but the truth is, the best exercise is whatever form of exercise you engage inconsistently. It really doesn't matter the form of exercise; if you don't engage in it regularly, you may not derive much benefit from it. That being said, you may find that engaging in high impact exercise is preferred—since you need not do them for very long to get major benefits. There are a variety of excellent immune-boosting workouts which last only 10 minutes or less available for free on the internet.

There are also great exercise apps you can download for free or inexpensively. Mossa Move is a popular one. Find whatever works for you. You might consider a prayer-walk partner. I love walking with my prayer-walk partners. A second wave of the pandemic is expected in the fall; the virus is here to stay. Engaging in short exercise creates a feeling of calm and equips you to handle adversity better which positions you to help those in need.

EXERCISE

This exercise provides a quick assessment of where you are today. We recommend that you repeat this check of your body, soul, and spirit wellness weekly every 30 days to see if you have moved up on the continuum. It doesn't matter where you start. What matters is that your current week's score is better than your last.

Ability to manage daily stress.	1 ☐	2 ☐	3 ☐	4 ☐	5 ☐	6 ☐	7 ☐	8 ☐	9 ☐	10 ☐
Consuming large amounts of fruit & vegetables	1 ☐	2 ☐	3 ☐	4 ☐	5 ☐	6 ☐	7 ☐	8 ☐	9 ☐	10 ☐
Exercising at least 30 minutes 3 times per week	1 ☐	2 ☐	3 ☐	4 ☐	5 ☐	6 ☐	7 ☐	8 ☐	9 ☐	10 ☐

Taking supplements daily	1 ☐	2 ☐	3 ☐	4 ☐	5 ☐	6 ☐	7 ☐	8 ☐	9 ☐	10 ☐
Avoiding drugs and reducing alcohol	1 ☐	2 ☐	3 ☐	4 ☐	5 ☐	6 ☐	7 ☐	8 ☐	9 ☐	10 ☐
Sleeping between 7 and 9 hours each night	1 ☐	2 ☐	3 ☐	4 ☐	5 ☐	6 ☐	7 ☐	8 ☐	9 ☐	10 ☐

Using relaxation techniques like the ones mentioned	1 ☐ 2 ☐ 3 ☐ 4 ☐ 5 ☐ 6 ☐ 7 ☐ 8 ☐ 9 ☐ 10 ☐

SCORE - WEEK 1	SCORE - WEEK 2
SCORE - WEEK 3	SCORE - WEEK 4

Chapter 5 - Mental and Emotional Thriving

I discussed ways to take care of your physical health in chapter four. I go into detail about how to maximize your mental, emotional, and spiritual well-being in this chapter. Of course, all parts of the self are inter-connected. For example, your physical health is connected to your emotional health. Therefore, try to engage in activities that apply to each aspect of your physical, emotional, mental, and spiritual well-being. You may wonder, "How do I have time to do all of this?" Good question! Incidentally, I'm swamped, so most of my methods take under thirty minutes.

Let's look at what causes us to feel overwhelmed. You may remember that after 9/11, there was an array of reactions from people around the country. Some were incapacitated and depressed for months, while others seemed fine a day or two later. Why such a difference? Well, a sense of humor helps. A sense of humor goes counts in challenging times, and a pandemic is one of those. There may be tough times ahead, given that people you know may not survive the pandemic. You or people you know may become sick or suffer financial losses, remember: some of the ideas in this book and prayer (if you are religious), can help deal with fear and grief.

It's natural to have feelings of fear, sadness, frustration, and anxiety during times of global and personal upheaval. When you feel such emotions, use effective outlets to release them— rather than taking them out on your household— or suppressing them. You may need to listen to music, or talk things through with someone you trust. You may need to let the tears flow or handle feelings of being overwhelmed with slow, deep breathing.

Remind yourself in such moments that this pandemic will pass. Painful moments will pass if you accept your feelings rather than deny them. Unfortunately, what you resist tends to persist. Thus, practice some of the techniques and advice in this book. Find effective ways to discharge uncomfortable feelings, so you don't startle or upset those around you. That may look like going for a run alone, with a running partner, or perhaps journaling.

I believe in having a sense of purpose or focus when dealing with challenging situations. If you're reading this book, you're well on your way! I want to give you a metaphor as to why some people respond to crises better than others. I'll use the metaphor of a tabletop to help you understand the varying reactions that people experience in crises. A table with a lot of legs is probably stable. A table needs a minimum of three legs to be stable; four is better, and any additional legs will simply add to its stability. If a table has only four legs, and two of those legs break, the table loses its support and collapses.

People who are equipped with adequate mental balance and psychological "legs" to stand on do better than those who do not, when the challenges come. What is a psychological "leg?" It is anything that helps you to feel Calm, Cared for, Connected, and/or in Control—the four C's. Think about it for a moment. The people who do well when dealing with life's stressors are those who have the four C's.

Let me give you an illustration. My father had diabetes during the last years of his life. The doctors periodically gave him dismal prognosis. Yet, because my Dad was skilled in finding inner calm, feeling cared for, and taking charge (a sense of control), he managed the stress very well. On the other hand, my family saw patients who were in better health than Dad when visiting him at the hospital, but were desperately unhappy and stressed. They lacked the ability to feel calm, cared for, connected, and in control.

Let's discuss how to incorporate each of 4 C's into your life, given that they are crucial for effectively managing crises. First, you must find ways to feel a sense of <u>Calm.</u> The important thing is that you find a method that works for you—and do it consistently. Common ways of finding calm include praying, yoga, tai Chi, massage, playing with pets, connecting with friends (perhaps over Zoom), listening to music, engaging in a creative project, reading, taking a relaxing bath, and meditation. Which of these ways of feeling calm have worked well for you in the past? Well, commit to doing them!

Think of your ability to tune into a feeling of peace and calm as an emotional bank account. If you frequently "invest" in such practices, your account "balance" will remain high. When disaster such as COVID-19 strikes, you will have "savings" in the bank which allows you make a withdrawal. People become emotionally depleted if they have little or no practice of contributing to their "calm account." The less investment they make in their calm account, the less able they are to handle crises because they have nothing to draw on. Do you know someone like that? Hopefully, it's not you—because it can be counterproductive.

The second C, is <u>Caring</u>. There are several ways to feel cared for. First, it helps to have people who care about you. Studies show that people who are quick to recover from trauma have close ties with friends and family. Such individuals also report being happier and healthier. Research suggests that people who have a few close relationships or no relationships may experience poor health. COVID-19 is forcing sheltering at home, and sometimes people are all alone. Call your friends, family members, and co-workers who are home alone. It will help to heal you and them. Do a Zoom or Skype call with them so you can feel even more connected. There's typically an increase in awareness of what really matters in life, based on what happened in China: people and not possessions. Unfortunately, people in the U.S.A work more hours than people in other developed nations. Of course, this results in higher standards of living. However, studies show that true happiness lies in our relationships with others, rather than how much money we have. No one has ever in their final moments of life said, "I wish I'd spent more time at my workplace." The more energy and time we invest in people we care about, the better able we are to cope with life's challenges, even pandemics.

The third "C" is <u>Connection</u>. What I mean by this is that you will benefit from establishing your connection to something bigger than yourself. Typically, that would be your connection with a higher power, for most of us, that is our relationship with God.   For some,   it's the connection to community or a charitable cause. Many people realized the importance of faith or spiritual connection after 9/11. I benefitted from a strong relationship with God and close relationships with other believers. We went for prayer walks, prayed together on the phone when we couldn't meet. I would encourage you to connect with a place of worship, whatever your faith may be.   Most faith-based organizations can conduct services online via zoom or skype, which makes it easier to connect. Your relationship with a higher power is something you draw upon in times of need, just like your "investment" in feeling calm and enjoying the people in your life.

When we have a sense of purpose and meaning, we can make sense of seemingly senseless things, as well as recover from trauma at a faster pace.

A sense of purpose and connection comes from being able to make valuable contributions to others. If you aren't already doing this, you might start by exploring your personal gifts are and what charity or causes you feel inclined to support. It feels good to contribute to a worthy cause. Contributing to one's world in a meaningful way helps create a greater sense of connection, as well as helping someone in need.

The last C stands for <u>Control</u>. Some personality types can maintain a semblance of control in almost any situation, whereas others feel completely out of control. What's the difference? It is a matter of perspective. For instance, young children cry when they are injured because they may not realize that the pain they are experiencing will eventually subside. Adults, on the other hand, know that things evolve, and nothing lasts forever. The higher the appreciation of this reality, the less likely we are to feel completely overwhelmed. We are in a unique position to create a plan for handling life's significant challenges—which is largely what this book is.

Corporate executives develop workable plans for responding to future catastrophes. Such plans build organizational confidence. Therefore, consider creating a list of short-term goals. Such a list would help combat feelings of anxiety that tend to follow during a crisis.

Most people do not like to write down goals, but I think you'll find this exercise so easy and beneficial that it'll be well worth the five minutes of effort it takes. Take out a piece of paper or create a document on your computer and title it, "Action Plan for Increasing the Four C's." (Or you can use the worksheet which follows this chapter). Next, write down the following questions, leaving a little space in between each question:

1. What small step can I take this week which will help me develop the ability to feel calm, peaceful, and at ease during these stressful times?

2. What small step can I take this week which will help me further develop a caring, intimate connection with my friends and family?

3. What small step can I take this week which will help me feel connected to some cause greater than myself?

4. What small step can I take this week which will help me to feel more in control of my life and/or my finances? Carve out a few minutes to answer these questions once you have put pen to paper. Think of a simple task that can easily be done within one week for each item. Once you make a note of it, place the piece of paper where you'll have a visual of it every day,

such as on your desk or refrigerator. You'll feel happier, healthier, and more in control, as you consistently take small steps towards increasing your ability with each "C."

The Three Minute Body Miracle

I discussed going from burned out to blissed out in the previous chapter. Would it be advantageous to learn how to do that? If your answer is in the affirmative, then the "Three Minute Body Miracle" (or T.M.B.M for short) is for you. According to the leading psychotherapist and creator of the technique, Jonathan Robinson, the amazingly effective four-step method does several things quickly. Robinson states that "*The technique gets your body naturally energized. Second, it stimulates blood flow to the brain for better focus and concentration. And finally, it lets you quickly let go of stress and tension in your body and mind. If you try it just a couple of times, I think you'll be hooked.*

First, since most people work once outside of the home (though more people are working from home due to the pandemic) and sit for long periods (as I do), step one is to stand up and shake your body. Our bodies were not meant to sit for long periods. It makes our joints hurt, and our muscles tighten. By shaking your shoulders, arms, legs, and hips for a mere one minute, you can stimulate energy and blood flow throughout your body. During your minute of shaking, make sure you vigorously move both your arms, shoulders, and legs. Pretend you're a rag doll, and you're able to shake the tension right out. You may feel embarrassed shaking your body vigorously for a full minute. If you are afraid of other people seeing you, close your office door, or go to the bathroom. Children move and shake all the time because it's a natural desire of our bodies to do so. Yet, as adults, we have become accustomed to being sedentary.

Unfortunately, not moving leads to feeling even more tired, which leads to even more lack of movement. Breaking this cycle is easier than you think. The main obstacles are complacency and fear of embarrassment. Since this entire process takes only three minutes (and only one minute of shaking), there's no good excuse for not doing it.

Second, imagine you're on a trampoline, and "bounce" up and down on your toes for thirty seconds. By doing this, you help counteract the force of gravity that can make you feel tired and stimulate your lymph glands and immune system. It's like giving your body an internal massage. The third step is to energetically massage your ears, face, and scalp for another thirty seconds. Your ears, face, and scalp are loaded with acupressure points that help to relax, energize, and balance your entire body.

Third, once you are done massaging your head, the last step is to take a very deep breath, tighten your shoulders by bringing them to your ears, and hold your breath for ten seconds. When you let go of your breath, exhale with a loud sighing sound as you feel the release of your shoulders. Focus for a moment on the feeling of warmth in your shoulders and face.

Finally, think of something or someone you feel grateful for. It could be your pet, your child, your health, your house, virtually anything. Feel a sense of gratitude in your heart for having this person, animal, or thing in your life. For a few moments, imagine you can breathe through your heart and have your gratitude expand with each breath. When you're ready, slowly open your eyes and notice how relaxed and energized you feel."

Try the above and see how that works for you. Once you strike that balance, you'll have a friend for life. Being able to tap into that positive energy releases endorphins into the system and boosts the immune system.

EXERCISE

Name three things you can engage in this week to help you feel a greater sense of <u>Calm</u>.

1. ____

2.

____

3.

____

Name someone who makes you feel <u>Cared</u> for and someone you can care for over the coming week.

I FEEL CARED FOR BY

I WANT TO CARE FOR

Now contact the person who has cared for you and thank them for their love and support.

What will you do to care for the person you identified above?

Name at least three areas where you feel you don't have control.

____

____

____

What small step can you take this week that will help you feel calm, peaceful, and at ease during this stressful time?

____

____

____

What small step can you take this week that will help you develop a caring, intimate connection with you friends and family?

____

____

____

What small step can you take this week that will help you feel connected to some cause greater than yourself?

____

____

____

What small step can you take this week that will help you to feel more in control of your life and/or your finances?

____

____

____

Take little but significant steps that leave you feeling revived, to increase your <u>Connection.</u> Perform one of the actions listed or ones that you think of over the week. Shade in the wheel, each time you do so. Try to fill up the wheel at least once each week.

<u>Suggestions</u>

Prayer

Meditation

Attend a spiritual gathering

Deep breathe

Hum/Sing

Volunteer

Donate to a charity

Perform this 3-minute challenge.

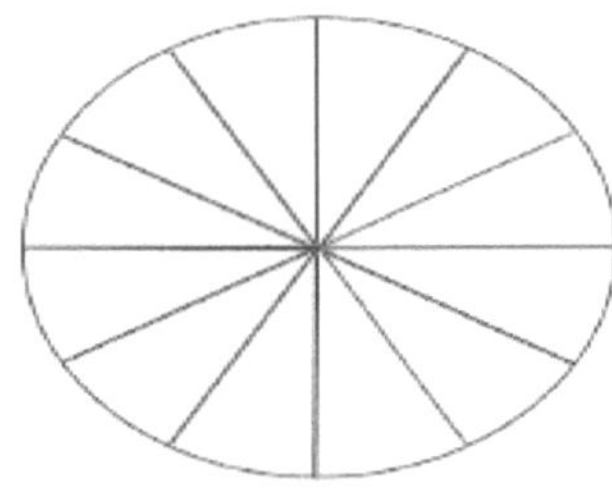

Excerpt from a newsletter contribution by Paula Anderson, a mental health professional on her work with college students during the pandemic:

"The following highlights the effects of COVID-19 on college students. Yes, they, too are finding ways to cope with the impact of the pandemic. How are college students and their mental health during COVID-19?

In my experience as a professional clinician and in speaking with several other colleagues, college students' experiences are varied, but some are experiencing a decline in their mental health. Do not get me wrong, many college students have fared well and are adjusting, but there are some who are having a difficult time managing the many changes. One in five students say their mental health has worsened during the coronavirus pandemic (Kerr, 2020). If you remember a long time ago (4 months back), these young people's freedom was ripped away from them as many of them, including my own young person, had to leave their dorms, apartments and college lifestyle within 24-72 hours. Some had a longer period, but the point is, things changed for them and changed quickly. With such a quick lifestyle change, many students were upset, stressed, and frustrated due to this change. What we know about change is that it can be met with resistance, fear, feelings of incompetence, and loss of identity. This is a lot to deal with as a student who has become used to a particular way of life. In one moment, they experienced several losses, such as loss of socialization, loss of college/college-life, and, like I mentioned before, loss of freedom.

The quick change not only interrupted their lifestyle disrupted the way they learn. Many of these students attended classes in person, looked forward to sitting with their peers in class, and had direct personal access to their professors. During the pandemic, they are forced to look at a screen all day, communicate with others through a chat feature, and have to take exams and finals in their bedrooms. This is no fun! Zoom fatigue is real- there are reports that state that being on videoconferencing is taking a toll on the brain and can be physically exhausting (Skylar, 2020).

I will highlight two other groups of college students who people may overlook. There are college students who come from abusive families and others who live in college housing because they are otherwise homeless. This group to me, are the ones that we should pay particular attention. The pandemic has forced some back into abusive households where their trauma is being triggered. Some mental health symptoms that they may experience are stress, anxiety, depression, and fear. For the college students who are homeless, they may experience the above symptoms and additionally must focus on necessities such as food, shelter, and finances.

As I pointed out, college students may be going through stress, loss/grief, anxiety, and depression over the many changes they have had to encounter over the past few months. College students are coping with these changes in both healthy and unhealthy ways. If you live with or have a college student in your midst, here are some ways to help:

If you notice any mental health symptoms such as chronic stress, anxiety, or depression, encourage them to seek virtual counseling. Typically they can receive counseling services through their colleges and universities, as well as through your insurance or using your company EAP benefits.

Encourage them to "hang" with their friends through FaceTime, and Zoom calls for ongoing social interaction. Chances are your social college student is already doing this. Encourage your student who may not be as social to connect with others.

For college students (who you are aware of) who may be in an unsafe home environment or may not have a steady place to live, encourage them to contact their college or university as they may have some options for summer housing or other community housing resources.

For college students who cope by being social and hanging with a lot of people, I will leave that up to you as to how you deal with this situation. However, just remember we have a responsibility to keep each other safe and to stop the spread.

Have some family fun, such as movie nights and game nights with your college student. Some young adults may not seem interested at first but do it anyway. Family bonding is so important."

Paula Anderson, is a Licensed Mental Health Clinician and Organizational Consultant in the Washington DC Metropolitan area. She is the founder of consulting firm, PACE Consulting (PACE), headquartered in College Park, MD. The organization specializes in delivering mental health counseling to children, adolescents, and adults, where we address concerns such as stress, anxiety, depression, relationship challenges, work stress, and career/life transitions. They also provide organizational consulting services that include management consulting, program development, staffing, and various training and workshops on workplace wellness. For more info on PACE, visit www.pace-consulting.com.

Chapter 6 - Helping Those You Care About

I mentioned in the previous chapter, that an excellent way to feel more fulfilled is to care for and contribute to the health and welfare of others. Of course, there are countless ways to do this. But before considering all the ways you may help your friends and family, please consider the advice you get on airplanes:

> "In case of emergency, air masks will drop from the ceiling. If you are traveling with a minor, please put on your own mask before helping the minor."

To most adults, the idea of putting on their own masks while a child or another vulnerable experiences discomfort right next to them may seem negligent. So why do airlines make this suggestion? Because if you are sick (or pass out due to lack of oxygen), you can no longer help those around you. So, your priority needs to be you. You must be in optimal shape to adequately care for others. Therefore your health and emotional wellbeing must come before anyone else's. That being said, once you feel adequately taken care of, there are a plethora of ways to help those you care about.

Think about creating new structures and routines. Has your daily routine been drastically altered? Perhaps your chilren are home since school are closed; perhaps you need to work from home or are now unemployed. How do you respond when suddenly presented with a lack of structure, or decimation of your daily routine? Do you become immobilized and shrink back or do you rise to the challenge and reinvent yourself? I encourage you to consider doing the latter! Create a new routine, a new normal and use it to your benefit in this time of crisis.

You may be wondering what that looks like, especially since you and your loved ones may not even be able to leave the house! Well, it will look different for every household, depending upon your resources, predilections, and creativity.

Below is a list of helpful ideas for creating some structure for you and your family:

1. Have your kids watch interesting, entertaining and educational videos at certain times of the day. You can simply Google "Educational videos for kids," ask the school for suggestions, or go to KhanAcademy.org for a list of videos.

2. Create artistic projects for yourself and your family. Once again, Google can be ☐uite helpful.

3. Carve out a specific time each day to go walking or move your body along with fitness videos on YouTube.

4. Keep to your routine of waking up and going to sleep at the same times each day.

5. Rethink activities that promote a sedentary lifestyle—such as an abundance of the TV or focus on media.

6. If you enjoy music or play an instrument, now is a great time to get some practice in.

7. Maintain a daily routine of prayer, meditation, or any other activity that nourishes your soul.

8. Read, read, and read some more! Commit to reading several pages of a great book daily.

9. Play board games with members of your household, or watch movies together.

10. If you are not working, think of creative ways to earn an income. There are so many ways to freelance and earn income in this day and age. Sites such as fiverr.com, upwork.com, and freelancer.com are great resources.

11. Now that you have extra time on your hands, consider learning a new skill such as how to cook, crochet, dance, build that she-shed you've always wanted, or learn how to play an instrument.

12. Set aside time to complete specific tasks like laundry, cleaning, or cooking. Use some of your time to attend to the emotional needs of loved ones. Take time to listen to fears or troubles of those around you without offering solutions. Bear in mind that when people express a need to talk, they're not necessarily looking for you to find a solution to their problems, they're just looking for an empathetic "listening ear." They want to be heard. The keyword is compassion and some more compassion! The pandemic has altered—and it will for while—the way we commune with friends and family. We can no longer be in their presence the way we were pre-pandemic. Fortunately, there are free video-conferencing services such as Facetime, Skype, Zoom, and

WhatsApp video. Zoom is great! They offer a free one to one video calls, and free group meetings that last less than 40 minutes. Zoom offers video chats with up to 99 for a fee. Look the information up if you haven't looked into it already.

You can also help those you care about by asking questions that engender positive feelings. It's easy to get overwhelmed with a barrage of bad news. A positive dialogue may alter a loved one's perspective for the better, while enhancing mood.

Here are ten questions that may help shift their focus to something other than loss, death, and ruin:

1. Did anything positive or good happen to you today? If so, what was it?

2. Is there anything you feel grateful for despite all that's things going on?

3. What act of kindness or help to others can you render or have rendered recently? If so, what did you do?

4. Have you seen any good movies or TV shows recently? If so, what was it and why did you like it?

5. What have you learned about yourself during this unusual time?

6. Is there anything I can do for you to help you during this challenging time?

7. What is something you appreciate about our connection?

8. Can you guess what I most appreciate about you? (Let them guess, and if they're wrong, tell them what you most appreciate).

9. Once this pandemic is over, do you think anything good will have come from it?

10. Has anything made you smile or laugh recently? If so, what was it?

You can ask someone all ten of these questions at once, depending on the circumstances, or just a single question per day. Once your friend or a family member answers a □uestion; you can respond to the same. If follow-up questions or dialogue arise from the answers, feel free to have them as well. It will bolster the relationship between you and your family member., We create moments of intimacy, when dialogue with loved ones. Such moments are both nourishing and healing. They can be game-changers!

It's important to maintain a positive attitude during this pandemic. We all know about the benefits of a positive attitude. I know what you're thinking. It's easier said than done, and I appreciate that. I can only encourage you to try. I want to offer a suggestion, and that is to try watching the following movies with your family members as a source of inspiration.   What follows is a list of the 15 most highly rated inspiring movies. Try Netflix or other similar resources.

Each of these movies can lift the spirits of you and your household:

1. War Room

2. Danjal

3. My Life as a Zucchini

4. Marriage story

5. Overcomer

6. Theory of Everything

7. Room

8. Fireproof

9. Same Kind of Different as Me

10. Her

11. Courageous

12. The Spectacular Now

13. Ralph Breaks the Internet

14. Silver Linings Playbook

Movies can be a great distraction and an excellent way to connect with members of your household. You can still enjoy watching a movie or TV show "together" by having your friend on the phone while you watch the same movie, even if you live alone.

In Case of Sickness

There's still a good chance you or someone you're close to may ultimately become sick, even though you put in your best effort. Experts predict that approximately half the world's population may get the virus before a vaccine is developed. Yikes! Okay, no need to panic should that happen. The good news is most people who contract the virus will recover. Common symptoms include (though scientists are still conducting studies to determine the full breadth of symptoms):

- Fever

- Shortness of breath

- Cough; and

- In the odd case, loss of sense of smell and taste.

- The above is by no means a complete list of *all* symptoms associated with the virus. Visit www.cdc.gov, www.nhs.uk, and www.who.int for updated information.

If you or a family member have any of the symptoms listed, call your healthcare provider. COVID-19 can be much more serious for individuals with underlying health conditions, such as diabetes and heart disease, are over 60 years of age, or have respiratory problems, such as asthma. While the overall death rate from the virus ranges from .7 % to 3% (depending on location), it is much higher for the elderly or those with compromised immune systems. However, new cases suggest that young people may also be at a higher risk of severe complications.

There is currently no treatment for the virus other than plenty of rest, fluids, Tylenol or paracetamol to reduce fever and further hospital care if necessary. Scientists are currently researching the efficacy of a common anti-inflammatory drug called Dexamethasone. The drug was once hailed as a ground-breaking therapy for those afflicted by the virus. We are yet to see the results of follow-up studies on the drug. However, we must tread with caution and follow advice from healthcare professional because there is so much that isn't known about this virus. That notwithstanding, there are many ways to assist family members who are sick with the virus. Get an N95 mask if a person you care for is sick, and maintain your distance and wash your hands frequently. The best thing you can do for you and a loved one is try not get infected.

I understand the plight of those who care for school-aged kids or aging parents. I'm sure you already had enough on your plate before the virus hit. Seek assistance from friends, family, neighbors, or anyone you know, to ensure you don't become completely overwhelmed. People rise to the occasion during unprecedented times.

Chapter 7 - Overcoming Pandemic-induced Trauma

Do you remember how you reacted to the events of 9/11? (9/11 is constantly referred to because the scale of devastation is almost comparable to what's happening with COVID-19). Your reaction, to some extent, depended on where you lived and whether or not you knew people who lost their lives that day. Yet, a major part of your reaction was due to your interpretation of the event, as well as your psychological preparedness for such a tragedy. Some people ended up being traumatized and depressed for months. They viewed the strike as the beginning of the end of the world or likened it to a major military action. On the other hand, other people saw it as an opportunity to pull together as a nation. The difference wasn't necessarily the amount of trauma they each experienced, but their reaction to it. I plan to share useful information in this chapter. The information will help you bounce back from whatever your reaction is or will be to this pandemic and future catastrophic events.

Much of the anxiety and emotional turmoil that occurs after a disaster stems from a feeling of helplessness. Fortunately, there are simple ways to regain a sense of hope. Once you feel more grounded, you'll be better equipped to handle the range of feelings and challenges that may follow.

People sometimes over-react once disaster strikes—thinking it's the end of the world. Remember that time eventually heals most wounds. Many people got upset all over again every time they watched the planes hit the twin towers. Yet , just as we all have the tendency to look at an accident on the side of the freeway, many people couldn't help but watch those terrible images again and again. Well, my advice is DON'T! When newscasters share data on coronavirus death and destruction, turn away. Better yet, use your radio to keep informed of what you need to know. It will save you a lot of grief, nightmares, and self-imposed trauma, because you can hear the information without seeing the images. More importantly, shield young children from such images. They are resilient in a different way. Their response to trauma sometimes has long-lasting effects. Stick with your daily routine as much as possible. Perform normal activities, such as cooking, laundry, housecleaning: it promotes calm and ease. Write tasks down, and create short-term goals. Maintain a visual of your to-do list: it will help you to stay focused.

Controlling Meaning

We often wonder why bad thing happens in life: we may not have the answers at first blush, but with the right perspective, we can process traumatic events effectively. The word "tragedy" signifies something terrible, but good things can materialize from tragic events. When the Japanese attacked Pearl Harbor, few Americans thought it was a good thing. Yet, looking back we can see that the attack led to the U.S. embarking on World War II quickly and more forcefully than we otherwise would have. The allies won the war and prevented more destruction and loss of life. My point is, when tragedy strikes, our reaction is typically based on the positive or negative meaning we attach to it and how wide or narrow our perspective is.

We sometimes attach the most disempowering interpretation when tragedy strikes. We say, "why me?" as if God is out to punish us, or we blame someone else or resort to victimhood. As a practicum, create your own positive and empowering interpretation of the event and ask yourself, what good could ultimately come. Such a question can be a major challenge to answer when disaster strikes. Yet, you must try.

Another question you might consider asking yourself soon after a tragedy is: "How can I respond to this event in a way that will lead to more inner strength, caring, and contribution to others?" You can counter feelings of powerlessness by contributing to the welfare of others, in the face of tragedy. You can empower yourself and others while creating a wholesome perspective.

A Pandemic (Economic) Depression

Two scenarios could unfold if the pandemic goes on longer than expected, or wreaks more havoc than is currently expected. The first (and more likely scenario) is that we will experience a recession for a period of 6 months to a couple of years. However, the worst-case scenario would look like the 1930's with actual price deflation, double-digit unemployment, and devastating economic losses globally.

The media may be saying the sky is falling, but ask yourself: "Is the worst actually happening?" You will have to make that determination yourself. The media may report that the financial markets are in complete meltdown, while Wall Street, the Feds, and the White House may attmept to "restore confidence" in the markets by delivering "feel-good" news. They may say upbeat things and avoid truths that are unpleasant. You must find information or advisors that are trustworthy and obtain reliable answers. Don't assume the worst.

Post-Traumatic Stress Disorder

According to the American Psychiatric Associaton, Post-Traumatic Stress Disorder (PTSD) is a psychiatric condition which manifests itself in people who personally witnessed or personally experienced a traumatic event. PTSD is an all-encompassing phrase for a predictable set of responses to major trauma. PTSD frequently leads to "recurring and intrusive" recall of the traumatic event or recurring and frightening dreams rehashing the event."

A diagnosis of PTSD requires manifestation of symptoms for at least a month after the initial event. 9/11 is an example of an event that induced PTSD in a lot of victims. Fortunately, there are effective treatments for PTSD. From complex psychological methods that require the expertise of a mental health professional to other proven techniques recognized by mental health experts. Symptoms of PTSD vary but fall into three main categories: hyperarousal, reexperiencing the event, and avoiding triggering situations. Here are some of the most common responses:

Hyperarousal, symptoms include difficulty sleeping, outbursts of anger, and lack of ability to focus. Signs that a person is re-experiencing the trauma include nightmares, intensely emotional, or physical reaction to reminders of the event and flashbacks. Finally, the third category, avoiding triggers, may include a person staying away from places, activities, people, or feelings related to the trauma, or feelings of detachment from people. Other more severe reactions are beyond the scope of this book.

If you or someone you love displays symptoms related to PTSD, first, realize it is common for people who have suffered trauma to experience PTSD-related symptoms. Second, seek help from a local therapist or online support group.

You can get helpful PTSD information and coping after disaster from the following web sites:

http://www.nimh.nih.gov (National Institute of Mental Health)

http://www.ptsdalliance.org (Posttraumatic Stress Disorder Alliance) or call them at (877) 507-PTSD

http://www.ncptsd.org (National Center for Post Traumatic Stress Disorder)

www.nhs.gov.uk (National Health Service UK)

Conventional treatments for PTSD include hypnotherapy and some new methods referred to as NLP and EMDR. You can ask a mental health professional if they are trained in any of these methods. The right treatment can alleviate the debilitating effects of PTSD.

The Erasure Technique is a method created by Psychotherapist, Jonathan Robinson. This technique is geared toward "erasing" bothersome memories stemming from traumatic events. Please note that this technique is not being offered in this book as treatment or therapy for any specific condition. The following is an excerpt from Robinson's work on "Finding Happiness."

Do bad memories or images ever haunt you? Do you sometimes flashback to some of the most traumatic moments of your past? The human mind has a tendency to forget important things like your mother's birthday but is more than happy to frequently remind you of your life's worst events. Fortunately, there's an antidote to this glitch in the human bio-computer. It's called the Erasure Technique. In a matter of a few minutes, this powerful method can virtually neutralize the bad feelings associated with almost anything you've ever experienced. I've even used it with clients who have suffered from disturbing memories for many years. Whether you want to neutralize images of a minor car accident or the hurt from the ending of a relationship, the erasure technique can make a dramatic difference. The theoretical underpinning of this method is that memories are stored in our brain in a similar way to how music is stored on a CD. Because precise information is encoded on a CD, every time you play it, it plays back the same music. But what if you took a nail and thoroughly scratched up the CD? If you tried to play it again, it wouldn't sound the same at all. In fact, your player would probably simply reject playing it. Well, in the Erasure Technique, something similar occurs. Using a precise process, we take a "nail" to your unpleasant memories and distort them until they are largely unrecognizable. Then, if you try to "play" the same memory again, your brain will either refuse to do so, or the memory will be so distorted that it will no longer have any impact on you. Voila! Your previously traumatic memory or image is neutralized.

Let's say you were once in a relationship where your partner said something incredibly hurtful to you, then walked out of your life. Of course, your brain thinks you need to see this scene several times a month, but you'd like to move on. You decide to use the erasure method. To do the technique, you begin by creating a "movie" of the event in your mind. You imagine the disturbing scene from the beginning, all the way to the very end. Yet, instead of watching it the way you normally do, play the scene in fast motion. When you get to the end of the "movie," play it in fast reverse. See all the characters moving very quickly, just like one of those early silent films.

Once you've watched the scene in fast forward and reverse, it's time to add a few props to the "movie." Imagine each and every person in the scene to be wearing a big pair of Mickey Mouse ears on their head. Then proceed to watch the unpleasant event in fast motion—forward and reverse—once again. Next, give everyone in the movie a gigantic red "Bozo" nose along with their Mickey Mouse ears. See the whole thing again in fast motion, forward and reverse. Finally, watch it at least one more time, this time adding circus music in the background and whatever ridiculous things your imagination can dream up. Once you've distorted the scene in these various ways, try to play your inner movie the way it used to be—the way it had tormented you before. What you'll likely notice is that ridiculous images keep "popping up" during the scene, even though you're not trying to create them. When your ex appears with Mickey Mouse ears and a Bozo nose, and their voice sounds like Daffy Duck as they speak to you, it's hard to take it all so seriously. Instead of a gut-wrenching feeling resulting from the memory, you'll feel pretty neutral about it. Congratulations! You've just healed yourself.

A client named Sharon came to me suffering from the fear of flying. When she was a little girl, she had been in a plane that made an emergency landing. She became terrified of getting on an aircraft. As luck would have it, her job required her to travel a lot. Occasionally she would "white knuckle" her way through a flight, but usually chose to drive—even if it was several hundred miles. I guided Sharon through the erasure process, focusing on both the original traumatic incident and recent times she had managed to get on a plane. She had fun picturing Mickey Mouse ears and Bozo noses on the flight attendants. She even laughed as she imagined clowns strolling down the aisles, complete with circus music, as the plane landed. As Sharon left my office, she was sure that such a simple process couldn't erase a lifetime of flying terror. Two weeks later, I got a call from her. After saying hello, Sharon told me she felt wonderfully relaxed. I asked her, "Is that unusual?" She responded, "You don't understand, I'm currently on an airplane, using one of those airplane phones! I feel no fear or anxiety at all. It worked!"

The erasure technique can be used for any sort of bothersome memory. In my practice, I've used it to help people who've suffered from flashbacks from accidents, embarrassing moments, and other adverse events and memories. In almost every case, after a few minutes of using this method a single time, the memory became much less bothersome. Occasionally, clients have to use the erasure technique a few times to get results, but it has always managed to help people feel better. If you have memories that still bother you or seem to have had a lasting negative impact on you, consider "erasing" them. By becoming more free of your past, it will be easier to create the future you truly desire."

This technique is quite frankly revolutionary. I gathered that it works so well that I decided to learn more about the author. However, like most techniques, the results or benefits can vary from person to person. What works for one person may not necessarily work for the other. If you are experiencing issues, explore the best options for you with your metal health provider.

Pandemic-induced Trauma

People all over the world are experiencing pandemic-induced trauma. They will need ways to cope, as the pandemic continues to unfold and people experience personal losses, such as death of loved ones, loss of livelihood, or are forced to stay at home for long periods. The following may help keep things in perspective and provide much-needed reassurance:

Are you prone to generalizing - engaging in broad negative conclusions while being trapped in a defeatist mindset?

Do you have an all or nothing view where everything is either black or white, or even absolute?

Are you quick to "look into a crystal ball" for predictions into the future and ultimately expect things to turn out wrong?

Are you prone to labeling yourself when you make mistakes and refer to yourself in less than flattering terms like, "I'm a loser," rather than, "I'm human, I made a mistake."

Do you downplay positive things in your life like your accomplishments and tell yourself they don't matter.

Do you engage in emotional reasoning while ignoring what the evidence suggests and tell yourself, "I feel like a failure, so everyone will now see me as a failure?"

Do you set unrealistic expectations and criticize others and yourself for not meeting them?

Do you make should've, could've, and would've statements rather than focusing on doing your best?

Now that you are more aware of some of your "thought errors," try the following exercise. Below is some room for you to write down common negative thoughts. Replace them with positive thoughts to help you to feel better.

PRACTICAL STEPS TO A MORE POSITIVE MINDSET

Example:

Limiting thought: I should have been more prepared for this.

I should have saved up more money for times like this.

New thought: No one could have predicted this was going to happen. I've been doing the best I can financially, and that's all I can do at this time. Everyone is going through a hard time; not just me.

Limiting thought: This awful feeling is just going to go on forever, and if I get the coronavirus, that will probably be the end for me.

New thought: Nothing lasts forever, I will feel much better once I get the help I need. Very few people die of the virus, but in all likelihood, I'd recover within a week or two.

<u>EXERCISE</u>

LIST ALL OF THE OLD LIMITING THOUGHTS YOU HAVE HAD

____

____

____

____

____

____

____

____

____

____

Now take each of those thoughts and write a positive response to each one.

Negative Thought

____

____

____

Positive thought

____

____

____

Negative thought:

____

____

____

Positive Thought:

____

____

____

Negative Thought:

____

____

____

Positive Thought:

____

____

Negative thought:

Positive Thought:

Negative thought:

Positive thought:

Negative thought:

Positive Thought:

Negative thought:

Positive Thought:

About the Author

Juliet Kika-Morrison is a social entrepreneur, who has a passion for pressing social issues, personal development, financial literacy, and physical wellness. Her entrepreneurial journey started with a partnership in a successful real estate title company in the DC metro area, which propelled her into solo practice for 7 years. Ms. Morrison made the transition from real estate during the economic crisis of 2008 to the education field which is also a passion of hers. She owned and operated a tutoring franchise until 2018 when she decided to pursue her doctorate. She holds a Law degree and a Master of Law degree. She is a 2022 candidate for a Doctor of Management in Organizational Development and Change. She is a change agent who has a passion for community organizing, social activism, creating business ventures, coaching, and public speaking. Her hobbies include travel, creating, and trying out new recipes and fine dining. When she is not working, she spends time in church fellowship, creating memories with her husband of 24 years and her daughter who is pursuing her undergraduate degree in the United Kingdom.

About the Contributing Author

Mr. Vincent Kika is a practicing NHS Emergency Medicine Consultant (Physician) in the UK. He is also a Clinical Negligence Solicitor (Lawyer) with a London firm. He is a Fellow of the Royal College of Surgeons and a Fellow of the College of Emergency Medicine. He obtained his LLB degree at the University of London and then completed the legal practice course at the College of Law, London, in 2008. Working as a doctor and a solicitor has afforded Dr. Kika the opportunity to develop his skills in the area of clinical negligence law with a number of transferable skills and a flexible and organized approach to work. He is an energetic, motivated, experienced, and dynamic team player. He takes a keen and active interest in clinical governance, quality of care delivered to patients, patient safety, and fairness for people affected by medical accidents.

Mr. Kika has practical knowledge and understanding of the law relating to clinical negligence litigation, the new NHS/private complaints procedure, the NHSLA Risk Management Standards for Acute Trusts and the Department of Health/Strategic health authority policy on health and patient's rights to receive a good quality of clinical care. He is passionate about justice and equality for all, particularly members of historically disadvantaged communities. As well as a strong work commitment, he has a keen interest in the development of legal and medical management softwares.